KIDNEY DISEASE DIET COOKBOOK

Essential Low-Sodium, High-Nutrient Recipes For Chronic Management And Renal Health

DR ELIAN GRIFFIN

DISCLAIMER

The nutritional recommendations and recipes in this book are meant solely for informative reasons. They are not meant to replace the counsel, diagnosis, or care of a qualified medical expert. If you have any doubts about a medical condition or dietary requirements, you should always see your physician or another trained healthcare expert.

All reasonable efforts have been taken by the author and publisher to ensure that the information contained in this book is correct as of the date of publication. Recommendations may alter, though, as medical knowledge is always changing. When using any of the recipes or instructions found here, the user assumes all liability and assumes no risk, whether personal or otherwise. People who have certain dietary requirements or medical issues should speak with a healthcare provider for personalized guidance. The given recipes are only ideas; you may need to adjust them to suit your own nutritional needs, tastes, and tolerances.

When you use this book, you agree to release the publisher, the author, and their representatives from any liability for any claims, damages, liabilities, costs, or expenditures resulting from your use of the book.

TABLE OF CONTENTS

ABOUT THE BOOK

The "Kidney Disease Diet Cookbook" is an invaluable tool for anyone attempting to manage kidney disease through dietary choices. Since diet has a direct impact on overall health and the efficacy of medical treatments, it is important to understand the critical role nutrition plays in kidney health. Renal nutrition, which is specifically designed to support kidney function, necessitates careful attention to essential nutrients like protein, sodium, potassium, phosphorus, and calcium, all of which are intricately balanced to maintain optimal health.

This cookbook is both a helpful reference and an extensive educational resource. It starts by describing the basic nutritional requirements for kidney health, stressing the significance of every nutrient in the effective management of the condition. From protein to vitamins, the cookbook offers insights into how these components contribute to balance and support renal function.

Meal prep for kidneys is made easier with specific strategies for creating balanced plates, portion control methods, and easy meal prep ideas. The advice also goes into grocery aisle navigation by highlighting ingredients that are appropriate for the renal diet so that shopping expeditions are in line with dietary needs.

From nutrient-dense breakfast options and flavorful main dishes to filling snacks and decadent desserts, the cookbook's pages contain a wide variety of carefully crafted recipes that are tailored to meet the varying meal times and preferences of kidney patients. Specific considerations, such as controlling sodium levels and customizing recipes for dialysis needs, are covered to provide readers with the knowledge they need to make educated culinary decisions.

Beyond recipes, the cookbook covers lifestyle considerations with strategies for staying active, handling dietary restrictions during social gatherings, and confidently navigating special occasions.

It also offers tips for maintaining optimal fluid balance, which is critical for kidney health.

The cookbook also includes answers to often-asked questions and concerns about things like protein consumption, managing fluids, and coping mechanisms for food cravings. It provides comfort and useful advice supported by medical knowledge.

Through the integration of culinary instruction and nutritional expertise, the "Kidney Disease Diet Cookbook" becomes an indispensable tool for anybody aiming to proactively manage their kidney health through a delightful and informed approach to eating.

CHAPTER ONE

KIDNEY DISEASE DIET INTRODUCTION

KIDNEY DISEASE OVERVIEW

Kidney disease, also referred to as renal disease, is a broad category of illnesses that impair the kidneys' capacity to remove waste products and extra fluid from the blood. This is an important function of the kidneys that helps maintain overall health because the kidneys also help control blood pressure, balance electrolytes, and produce hormones necessary for bone health and red blood cell production.

Acute kidney injury (AKI) is an abrupt condition brought on by dehydration, infection, or medication side effects. Both CKD and AKI require careful management to avoid complications and maintain kidney function.

To maintain quality of life, it is important to understand kidney disease and its various stages, which range from mild impairment to complete kidney failure requiring dialysis or transplantation. Early detection through routine screenings is crucial because symptoms may not appear until significant kidney damage has occurred. Treatment focuses on treating the underlying causes of kidney disease, managing symptoms, and implementing lifestyle changes, such as dietary modifications that support kidney health.

The holistic management of kidney disease includes medical treatment, dietary changes, and lifestyle modifications. People who are aware of the basic principles of kidney function and disease progression can take an active role in their care, working with healthcare providers to improve overall health and optimize outcomes.

DIET IS CRUCIAL FOR MANAGING CHRONIC KIDNEY DISEASE

A kidney-friendly diet focuses on controlling the intake of certain nutrients like sodium, potassium, phosphorus, and protein, which can accumulate to harmful levels when kidney function is impaired.

Monitoring these elements through dietary modifications can help maintain a balance that supports kidney function and overall health. Dietary management is crucial for managing kidney disease because it can help reduce symptoms, slow down the progression of the disease, and reduce complications.

Understanding how different foods affect blood chemistry and kidney function is essential to renal nutrition. For example, controlling blood pressure and sodium intake helps prevent electrolyte imbalances and mineral buildup that can eventually harm kidney function; controlling potassium and phosphorus intake helps prevent mineral buildup and electrolyte imbalances; controlling protein intake helps control blood waste products, which reduces kidney stress and supports optimal kidney function.

A customized diet plan considers a person's nutritional requirements, medical history, and stage of kidney disease. Speaking with a registered dietitian with expertise in renal nutrition can offer individualized advice, guaranteeing that dietary changes are both sustainable and successful. People who adopt a kidney-friendly diet can improve their overall health, reduce complications related to kidney disease, and improve their quality of life.

FUNDAMENTALS OF NUTRITION FOR THE RENAL SYSTEM

Renal nutrition is centered on optimizing dietary choices to support kidney health and effectively manage kidney disease. Important concepts include limiting the intake of nutrients such as potassium, sodium, phosphorus, and protein—all of which are essential for kidney function and general health—and understanding the interactions between these nutrients and the body's chemistry to help people make more informed dietary decisions and promote proactive management of kidney disease.

It is critical to monitor potassium levels, particularly in advanced stages of kidney disease, to prevent abnormal heart rhythms and muscle weakness. Phosphorus management involves limiting intake to prevent bone and cardiovascular complications associated with high levels in the blood. Protein moderation aims to reduce the burden on kidneys tasked with filtering waste products, promoting kidney function preservation. Sodium restriction is crucial in renal nutrition because excess sodium can lead to fluid retention and elevated blood pressure, straining the kidneys.

By following a customized nutrition plan, people can optimize their dietary habits, lower the complications associated with kidney disease, and enhance their quality of life. Renal nutrition enables people to take an active role in managing their health through dietary choices that support kidney function and overall well-being.

HOW YOU CAN USE THIS COOKBOOK TO HELP

With its practical advice and delicious recipes designed to support kidney function and promote overall wellness, this kidney disease diet cookbook is a great tool for anyone navigating the challenges of managing their kidney health through nutrition.

Each recipe is meticulously crafted to adhere to renal nutrition guidelines, with a focus on nutrient balance and portion control to meet the unique dietary needs of people with kidney disease.

Whether someone is looking to manage kidney disease in its early stages or needs dietary adjustments for more advanced conditions, this cookbook offers a variety of flavorful dishes that satisfy different palates and dietary preferences while still adhering to recommended nutritional guidelines.

It also makes kidney disease diet maintenance easier with its satisfying and nutritious recipes that don't sacrifice taste.

In addition to recipes, the cookbook offers educational content on renal nutrition that explains the underlying principles of dietary recommendations and how they help effectively manage kidney disease. It gives people the power to make educated diet decisions and supports them in taking charge of their health and improving their overall quality of life by adopting healthy eating habits.

<h2 style="text-align:center">USING THE RECIPES AND INSTRUCTIONS</h2>

Each recipe in this cookbook comes with clear instructions, ingredient lists, and nutritional data so that readers can make educated meal choices and track their intake of important nutrients. The recipes and guidelines are organized in an easy-to-use format so that people can easily incorporate kidney-friendly meals into their daily routines.

In addition to encouraging creativity in meal planning while adhering to renal nutrition principles, the cookbook offers flexibility by providing recipes appropriate for various meal times and occasions, ranging from hearty main dishes to satisfying snacks and desserts. This empowers individuals to enjoy a varied and flavorful diet that supports kidney health.

Follow the guidelines in the cookbook and people can confidently navigate their way towards better kidney health, one delicious meal at a time. The cookbook includes recipes as well as helpful tips and tricks for meal preparation, storage, and ingredient substitutions, making it easier to adapt recipes to individual preferences and dietary needs.

CHAPTER TWO

CRUCIAL ELEMENTS FOR HEALTHY KIDNEYS

AN OVERVIEW OF THE REQUIREMENTS FOR NUTRITION

To manage and prevent kidney disease, it is imperative to have a thorough understanding of the nutritional requirements for kidney health.

The main goals of a kidney-friendly diet are to balance protein intake, control sodium and potassium levels, regulate phosphorus and calcium intake, and maintain adequate hydration without overloading the kidneys with fluid. The exact nutritional requirements of each individual will depend on the stage of kidney disease, other medical conditions, and treatment plans.

A diet rich in fruits, vegetables, whole grains, and lean proteins is generally associated with kidney health; processed foods high in sugar and sodium should be avoided; eating a diet rich in fresh, unprocessed foods promotes overall health and a balance of nutrients;

cooking with baking, grilling, or steaming is a healthier way to cook than frying.

For people with kidney disease, it's important to keep an eye on portion sizes and be aware of the nutritional value of foods. It's also advisable to meet with a dietitian or healthcare provider regularly to create customized diet plans that meet individual needs. These personalized approaches can help manage symptoms, prevent complications, and enhance quality of life.

THE VALUE OF SODIUM, POTASSIUM, AND PROTEIN

Lean meats, fish, eggs, and dairy products are high-quality protein sources that provide essential amino acids while minimizing waste products that the kidneys must filter out. However, excessive protein intake can worsen kidney damage, so it's important to find the right balance based on individual health needs and kidney function. Protein is an essential nutrient for overall health, but for those with kidney disease, the type and amount consumed must be carefully monitored.

Sodium is an important component of blood pressure regulation and fluid balance. People with kidney disease should minimize their sodium intake to avoid fluid retention and high blood pressure, both of which can deteriorate kidney function.

This includes cutting back on the amount of table salt that they use, avoiding packaged and processed foods, and flavoring meals with fresh herbs and ingredients instead of table salt. It's also important to read food labels and be aware of hidden sodium in condiments and restaurant meals.

The kidneys regulate potassium levels, and impaired kidney function can result in an accumulation of potassium in the blood.

To manage potassium levels, it's important to be aware of high-potassium foods like bananas, oranges, potatoes, and tomatoes, and to balance their intake with other lower-potassium options. Regular monitoring of blood potassium levels can help guide dietary choices and prevent complications.

Potassium is necessary for muscle function and heart health, but too much of it can be dangerous for those with kidney disease.

RECOGNIZING THE BALANCE OF PHOSPHORUS AND CALCIUM

High phosphorus levels can cause weakened bones and other health problems, so it's important to limit foods high in phosphorus, like dairy products, nuts, seeds, and certain processed foods. Instead, choose lower-phosphorus alternatives like rice milk, non-dairy creamers, and certain fruits and vegetables. Phosphorus is a mineral that helps build strong bones and teeth, but maintaining phosphorus levels in people with kidney disease can be challenging.

A dietitian can assist in developing a diet plan that guarantees adequate calcium intake while controlling phosphorus levels. Calcium supplements or high-calcium foods need to be consumed with caution to avoid further complicating the phosphorus-calcium balance.

Calcium is equally important for bone health, but its relationship with phosphorus must be carefully balanced. When phosphorus levels are high, calcium can be pulled from the bones, weakening them.

To maintain the proper balance and support overall kidney health, managing the phosphorus and calcium balance often entails the use of phosphate binders; medications that help prevent the absorption of phosphorus from foods. To be effective, these medications are usually taken with meals and snacks. Regular monitoring of blood levels and dietary and medication plans accordingly can help maintain the right balance.

TIPS FOR FLUID MANAGEMENT

Controlling fluid intake is critical for people with kidney disease because it keeps the kidneys from being overworked and prevents complications like swelling, hypertension, and heart problems. Depending on the stage of the disease and the existence of other conditions like heart failure, there are differences in how much fluid an individual should drink. Generally speaking, this means keeping an eye on everything that contains water, including drinks and foods like soups, fruits, and vegetables.

Using smaller cups and glasses to help control the amount of liquid consumed is one useful tip for managing fluid intake; another is to sip fluids gradually throughout the day instead of consuming large amounts at once; tracking daily fluid intake with a journal or an app can help stay within recommended limits.

It is helpful to avoid high-sodium foods, which can increase thirst, chew gum, suck on ice chips, or use mouthwash to keep the mouth moist to reduce thirst and control fluid intake.

Additionally, routine check-ups with a healthcare provider can help customize fluid intake recommendations based on individual health needs and kidney function.

Minerals and vitamins are necessary for good health overall, but people with kidney disease may need to modify their vitamin and mineral intake. For example, water-soluble vitamins (Vit C, and B vitamins) are generally advised because they are excreted in urine and are not stored in the body; they boost energy, the immune system, and general health.

On the other hand, fat-soluble vitamins (Vit A, D, E, and K) must be taken with caution to prevent toxicity.

Another essential mineral is iron, which is particularly important for people with kidney disease who may experience anemia. Iron-rich foods such as beans, lean meats, and fortified cereals can help you maintain healthy iron levels; in certain circumstances, you may need to take iron supplements under a doctor's supervision. Making sure you get enough vitamin C can also help your body absorb iron from plant-based sources.

Regular blood tests can provide insights into nutrient levels and guide dietary adjustments. Calcium and magnesium are essential for bone health and muscle function, but their levels must be carefully balanced. People with kidney disease often need to monitor their intake of these minerals to prevent complications. A dietitian can help identify appropriate food sources and supplements to ensure that all necessary vitamins and minerals are included in the diet without overloading the kidneys.

CHAPTER THREE

BUILDING BALANCED MEALS

Developing a kidney-friendly diet requires thoughtfully choosing foods that are low in sodium, potassium, and phosphorus while still providing enough protein. Begin with a foundation of whole grains, such as quinoa or brown rice, which offer fiber and important nutrients without adding too much phosphorus. Combine this with lean protein sources, like fish or chicken breast, which are lower in potassium than red meats. Add a range of vibrant vegetables, such as carrots, kale, and bell peppers, which are high in vitamins and minerals but low in potassium.

Use spices and herbs like garlic powder, turmeric, or basil to enhance flavor without adding sodium. Finally, add a small amount of healthy fats from avocado or olive oil to support overall nutrient absorption. By balancing these ingredients, you can make nutritious, filling meals that promote kidney health without sacrificing taste.

TIPS FOR PORTION CONTROL

Using smaller plates can help visually control portions and prevent overeating. Fill half of your plate with non-starchy vegetables, a quarter with lean protein, and the remaining quarter with whole grains or starchy vegetables. Portion control is important in managing kidney disease because it helps regulate the intake of nutrients that can impact kidney function.

To properly portion foods higher in potassium or phosphorus, like dairy products or bananas, use measuring cups or a food scale. You should also be aware of the amount of liquid you drink, choosing water instead of sugary drinks to stay hydrated without consuming extra calories or phosphorus. By following these guidelines, you can effectively manage the health of your kidneys while eating balanced meals that satisfy your nutritional needs.

Planning your meals ahead of time and selecting recipes low in sodium, potassium, and phosphorus are good ways to ensure that you have kidney-friendly meals available throughout the week. You can also batch-cook proteins, such as baked fish or grilled chicken, and then portion them out into individual servings for easy reheating.

Meal prep ahead of time to save time on busy days and maintain a consistent diet that supports kidney health. Prepare grains and vegetables that can be kept in the fridge or freezer, like quinoa salad or roasted vegetables, to go with your main dishes. Store meals in portioned containers so they're easy to grab and go for work or outings. Label containers with instructions on how to reheat food to ensure proper food safety and quality.

RENAL DIET GROCERY SHOPPING

When grocery shopping, choose foods low in sodium, potassium, and phosphorus, with an emphasis on whole, fresh ingredients. Make a list based on the meals you plan to prepare each week, emphasizing fresh fruits and vegetables (such as apples, berries, and green beans) that are lower in potassium. Select lean protein sources (like eggs or poultry) and steer clear of processed meats that are high in sodium.

You can maintain a well-rounded diet that supports your overall health by planning your grocery trips around kidney-friendly foods. Choose whole grains like oats or barley, which provide fiber without adding excess phosphorus. Carefully read food labels to avoid products with added sodium or phosphorus-based additives. Consider shopping in the perimeter of the grocery store, where fresh produce and unprocessed foods are typically located.

RECIPES FOR VARIOUS MEAL TIMES

Planning kidney-friendly dishes for various meal times will help you eat well and taste good all day. For breakfast, consider a low-potassium fruit smoothie made with yogurt, berries, and a tiny bit of protein powder. For lunch, think about a mixed green salad with grilled chicken and a vinaigrette dressing made with herbs and olive oil.

Dinner should be baked fish served with quinoa and seasoned steamed vegetables. Nuts and low-sodium crackers with hummus are good snack options. Experiment with different herbs and spices to add flavor without adding sodium or phosphorus. By trying out different recipes that are customized to your dietary needs, you can eat a varied and fulfilling diet that promotes kidney health.

CHAPTER FOUR

MEAL PLANNING: BREAKFAST RECIPES

IDEAS FOR LOW-PROTEIN BREAKFASTS

A low-protein diet is often advised for people with kidney disease to reduce the strain on the kidneys and effectively manage symptoms. One way to create a low-protein breakfast that is both satisfying and nutritious is to substitute low-protein foods for high-protein ones, such as eggs and meats.

For example, you can start your day with a bowl of oatmeal made with water or a plant-based milk substitute, top it with fresh berries, and add a dash of flaxseed or chia seeds for extra fiber and omega-3s. Alternatively, you can make a smoothie that combines low-protein fruits, like apples or pears, with spinach or kale for extra nutrients.

For a variety of low-sodium, low-potassium breakfast options, try combining whole grain toast spread with a small amount of avocado or nut butter with a side order of fresh fruit or a small serving of low-potassium vegetables such as bell peppers or cucumbers; if you prefer a warm breakfast, make a vegetable and rice porridge seasoned with herbs and a little olive oil; this will ensure that it is low in potassium and sodium.

SHAKES & SMOOTHIES FOR PATIENTS ON DIALYSIS

Smoothies and shakes are an easy way for dialysis patients to get more nutrients without going overboard with protein, potassium, or phosphorus. To keep phosphorus levels in check, start with a base of low-potassium fruits like berries, apples, or pineapples blended with nondairy milk like almond or rice milk. Add a handful of spinach or kale for extra vitamins and minerals. If your doctor suggests it, add a scoop of low-protein protein powder.

If you would like your shakes to be thicker, then blend in half an avocado or a frozen banana, which adds creaminess without sacrificing nutritional value. If you would like your shakes to taste better, then add a small amount of vanilla or cinnamon extract, which can add flavor and aroma without using any salt or sugar. These shakes can be consumed as a quick breakfast or as a convenient kidney-friendly snack.

OPTIONS FOR HIGH-CALORIE BREAKFASTS

Those with kidney disease may find it difficult to consume enough calories, particularly when undergoing dialysis. However, high-calorie breakfast options can help satisfy daily energy requirements without taxing the digestive system or sacrificing dietary restrictions. For starters, try starting with a bowl of whole-milk oatmeal or a plant-based milk substitute that has been fortified with extra nutrients.

On top of it, add nuts or seeds for extra calories and healthy fats, and drizzle with honey or maple syrup for sweetness.

A whole-grain tortilla stuffed with scrambled eggs or tofu, black beans, avocado, and salsa makes a breakfast burrito that offers a well-balanced combination of protein, healthy fats, and carbohydrates to keep you feeling energized all morning. If you'd rather have something lighter, a parfait consisting of layers of yogurt, fresh fruit, and a dollop of nut butter is a filling but high-calorie option that will make sure people with kidney disease get enough calories to support their daily activities and general health.

EASY AND QUICK BREAKFAST RECIPES

Making quick and simple breakfasts is crucial when dealing with the symptoms of kidney disease. Choose low-preparation foods that are quick to put together and don't compromise on nutrition. One popular option is overnight oats, which are made by putting oats, milk or yogurt, chia seeds, and fruits in a jar and refrigerating overnight to have breakfast ready in the morning. Another option is to make a batch of egg muffins with cheese and veggies that can be made ahead of time and then reheated whenever necessary during the week.

Smoothie bowls made with blended fruits, yogurt, or milk, and a variety of toppings like nuts, seeds, and coconut flakes offer a refreshing and customizable breakfast option. These quick meals ensure individuals with kidney disease can start their day with a nutritious and satisfying meal that supports their dietary needs and busy lifestyle. For a lighter option, Greek yogurt topped with granola and fresh berries provides a balance of protein, fiber, and vitamins without requiring any cooking.

HOW TO IMPROVE FLAVOR WITHOUT ADDING SODIUM

For those with kidney disease, flavor enhancement without sodium is essential because too much salt can aggravate symptoms. Try using herbs and spices like turmeric, thyme, and basil to give dishes more flavor and complexity without adding more sodium. You can also play around with citrus juices like lemon or lime to enliven flavors and bring dishes to balance without adding salt.

These suggestions ensure that meals are flavorful and enjoyable while supporting kidney health by minimizing sodium intake. Grill or roast vegetables to bring out their natural sweetness and enhance their texture; add a little olive oil and herbs for flavor; use vinegar- or mustard-based dressings in salads or as marinades for meats to provide tanginess and depth without adding salt; use dried or fresh herbs in cooking instead of pre-packaged seasoning mixes, which are frequently high in sodium.

DIABETIC-FRIENDLY MAIN COURSES

To make kidney-friendly main dishes, start with ingredients and cooking techniques that promote kidney health. Lean proteins, like fish, chicken, or turkey, are less taxing on the kidneys than red meats.

To reduce fat content and enhance flavor without adding extra sodium, marinate your protein of choice in a mixture of olive oil, lemon juice, garlic, and herbs like rosemary or thyme. Finally, bake or grill the protein rather than fry it.

Add lots of low-potassium veggies, like bell peppers, cabbage, cauliflower, and green beans. You can roast or steam these veggies and add some extra flavor by drizzling them with olive oil and sprinkling some herbs on them. To make a full meal, combine your protein and veggies with a small amount of whole grains, like couscous or quinoa, which are lower in phosphorus and potassium than brown rice or whole wheat products.

Try different kidney-friendly seasonings and sauces to add variation. Store-bought sauces often contain high levels of salt and phosphorus; make your kidney-friendly sauces to maintain ingredient control and kidney-friendliness.

A simple lemon herb sauce made with lemon juice, olive oil, garlic, and fresh herbs can elevate your dish without adding extra sodium.

OPTIONS FOR VEGETARIANS AND VEGANS

Kidney-friendly vegetarian and vegan diets are abundant and high in nutrients. When preparing these plant-based proteins, use minimal amounts of salt and flavor-enhancing herbs and spices like cumin, coriander, and turmeric. Plant-based proteins low in potassium and phosphorus include tofu, tempeh, and legumes like lentils and chickpeas.

Add a rainbow of vibrant, low-potassium veggies, like bell peppers, cauliflower, zucchini, and eggplant; these can be roasted, grilled, or stir-fried with garlic and olive oil for a tasty, kidney-safe supper. Fresh herbs, like basil, parsley, and cilantro, can enhance the flavors and provide extra nutrition without adding extra salt.

Grains such as quinoa, bulgur, and barley make great foundations for kidney-friendly vegetarian and vegan recipes. Toss them with your favorite veggies and plant-based proteins for a well-balanced meal.

To add some taste, try preparing a simple dressing of olive oil, lemon juice, garlic, and herbs to drizzle over your dish right before serving.

SIDES AND SALADS LOW IN POTASSIUM

Choosing the right ingredients and dressings is key to making tasty, low-potassium salads and sides. Start with a base of low-potassium greens, like iceberg lettuce, romaine, or arugula, then add a variety of colorful, crunchy vegetables, such as bell peppers, cucumbers, radishes, and cabbage, which add texture and nutrients without adding a lot of potassium.

Add a little bit of low-potassium protein-boosting ingredients to your salad, such as cooked chicken, tofu, or boiled eggs; for dressings, make a basic vinaigrette with olive oil, apple cider vinegar, lemon juice, and your favorite herbs and spices; this will keep your salad tasting great and not too high in sodium or potassium.

Low-potassium ingredients can also help make side dishes kidney-friendly. Try roasting or steaming veggies like cauliflower, carrots, and green beans; toss them with olive oil, garlic, and herbs for extra flavor. Alternatively, make a grain-based side like white rice or couscous mixed with chopped vegetables and a light dressing; this makes a healthy and delicious side to your main dish.

CONTROLLING SODIUM IN TASTY RECIPES

For the sake of kidney health, cut back on sodium in savory dishes by choosing recipes that use herbs, spices, and citrus flavors instead of salt. For instance, make a homemade vegetable soup seasoned with garlic, thyme, and a squeeze of lemon juice to brighten the flavors.

This will minimize sodium content while maximizing taste and nutrition. Another tactic is to marinate meats in citrus juices and herbs before grilling or baking, which adds depth of flavor without going overboard. Finally, when making pasta dishes, make homemade tomato sauce with fresh herbs and garlic instead of pre-made sauces that are high in sodium and additives.

ONE-POT DINNERS FOR SIMPLE CLEANING

The convenience of one-pot meals extends to kidney-friendly options as well. One popular option is chicken and vegetable stir-fry, which combines lean chicken breast, colorful vegetables, and low-sodium soy sauce in one pan. This dish is easy to make and requires little cleanup. Another tasty option is shrimp and vegetable quinoa pilaf, which is cooked with aromatic vegetables and seasoned with herbs for a full meal in one pot. Finally, for a hearty and kidney-friendly dinner, try turkey chili, which is made with lean ground turkey, kidney beans, and diced tomatoes and seasoned with cumin and chili powder.

You can create delicious dishes that support kidney health without sacrificing taste or variety by focusing on fresh, low-phosphorus, low-potassium, and low-sodium ingredients. These recipes and meal ideas offer doable solutions for incorporating kidney-friendly ingredients while maintaining flavor and nutrition.

HEALTHY SNACKS FOR PEOPLE WITH KIDNEY DISEASE

Choosing low-sodium, low-potassium, and low-phosphorus foods that still contain vital nutrients is a good way to find healthy snacks for kidney patients. Here are some examples: try cinnamon-sprinkled apple slices for flavor without adding extra sodium; air-popped popcorn for a low-phosphorus and low-sodium snack that satisfies cravings without harming kidney health; and Greek yogurt with fresh berries for protein and antioxidants that is lower in potassium than other dairy products.

When making snacks, homemade options such as hummus-topped vegetable sticks offer fiber and protein without the high sodium content of many prepackaged dips.

Similarly, rice cakes with a small amount of almond butter provide a crunchy texture and a protein boost without being overly phosphorus-rich.

By selecting these snacks, kidney patients can indulge in delicious foods while following dietary guidelines that promote their general well-being.

OPTIONS WITH LOW PHOSPHORUS

Controlling phosphorus intake is important for kidney patients because high phosphorus intake can cause problems. Fresh fruits (apples, grapes, strawberries) and vegetables (bell peppers, cucumbers, carrots) are good examples of low-phosphorus snacks. Hard-boiled eggs are a good protein source and a low-phosphorus snack because they are naturally low in phosphorus.

When it comes to snacks, unsalted rice cakes with avocado slices and a dash of sesame seeds are a great option because they provide fiber, healthy fats, and a satisfying crunch without the phosphorus that many other snack options have.

As for drinks, try herbal teas or homemade lemonade sweetened with a sugar substitute to avoid getting extra phosphorus.

Kidney patients can better control their phosphorus levels and support kidney function by including these low-phosphorus options in their daily snack routines.

FAST APPETIZERS FOR PARTICULAR EVENTS

The right recipes make it easy and fun to prepare quick appetizers for special occasions while following a kidney-friendly diet. One such recipe is cucumber rounds topped with a small dollop of low-sodium cream cheese and a sprinkle of dill; this refreshing appetizer is low in sodium and adds a flavorful burst to any gathering. Another popular appetizer is bruschetta, which is made with diced tomatoes, basil, and a drizzle of balsamic vinegar on whole-grain toast; this dish is high in antioxidants, has a satisfying crunch, and is low in phosphorus and sodium.

Prepare skewers of grilled chicken or tofu with colorful bell peppers and cherry tomatoes for a protein-rich appetizer. These skewers are simple to put together and pair well with a kidney-friendly yogurt and herb dipping sauce. When preparing appetizers for special occasions, emphasize using fresh ingredients and straightforward preparations so that everyone can enjoy delectable snacks that promote kidney health.

TIPS FOR PORTION CONTROL IN SNACKING

Kidney patients must practice portion control to manage their nutrient intake and prevent overconsumption of sodium, potassium, and phosphorus.

Pre-portioned snacks, such as single-serving packs of unsalted rice cakes or low-sodium popcorn, can help reduce cravings while simplifying portion control. Because nuts and pretzels can be high in sodium, measure your snack intake to avoid going over the recommended serving sizes.

In addition, mindful snacking—which involves paying attention to hunger cues and stopping when full instead of eating until satisfied—helps individuals avoid overindulging and promotes kidney health by keeping a balanced diet. People can also enjoy snacks throughout the day without sacrificing their nutritional objectives by portion controlling and choosing kidney-friendly snacks.

WHOLESOME SPREADS AND DIPS

Producing tasty and nutritious dips and spreads for individuals with kidney disease requires selecting ingredients that are low in sodium, potassium, and phosphorus. For example, mashed avocado, lime juice, and a small amount of salt substitute can be combined to make a creamy, kidney-friendly guacamole dip. This dip pairs well with raw vegetable sticks, such as cucumber, celery, and bell peppers, and makes a filling, vitamin- and fiber-rich snack. Chickpeas, garlic, and olive oil can be blended until smooth to make hummus, which is high in protein and fiber and low in phosphorus and sodium.

To make a nutrient-dense snack that is dairy-free, blend silken tofu with lemon juice, garlic, and herbs to make a creamy tofu spread.

This spread can be used as a dip for whole-grain crackers or as a topping for sliced vegetables. To keep kidney health in check when making dips and spreads, use fresh ingredients and minimize added salt. Kidney patients can benefit from tasty options that support their dietary needs by including these healthy dips and spreads in their snack times.

DESSERTS WITH LESS SUGAR FOR A KIDNEY DIET

When it comes to making sweet treats that still taste good and follow a kidney-friendly diet, one way to do this is to use natural sweeteners like stevia or monk fruit, which provide sweetness without raising blood sugar levels. Another way is to use fruits like berries, which have less sugar than other fruits but still taste sweet and naturally sweet.

Lastly, adding unsweetened applesauce or mashed bananas can improve sweetness and moistness in baked goods without requiring added sugars.

For example, here's a low-sugar berry parfait recipe: layer fresh berries with a Greek yogurt mixture sweetened with a little honey or vanilla extract. This dessert gives you both protein and probiotics, which makes it a nutritious option for kidney health. If you're in the mood for something warm and comforting, try this baked apple dessert dusted with cinnamon and nutmeg. By making these choices, people can enjoy desserts guilt-free while supporting their kidney health goals.

FRUIT-BASED DESSERTS

Because fruits contain less potassium and phosphorus than many other dessert ingredients, they are an essential part of a kidney-friendly diet. Fruit-based desserts provide a naturally sweet and refreshing taste without violating dietary restrictions. For example, a simple fruit salad with apples, grapes, and melons offers a medley of flavors and textures that is ideal for sating a sweet tooth. Alternatively, blending frozen bananas with a little almond milk makes a rich and satisfying "nice cream," a healthier take on traditional ice cream.

In addition, adding fruits to desserts such as grilled peaches or mango salsa enhances flavors and offers a fulfilling way to conclude a meal. These desserts not only support kidney health but also provide essential vitamins, minerals, and antioxidants that are important for general health.

Through experimenting with various fruits and preparation techniques, people can find delicious dessert options that complement their kidney health journey.

KID-FRIENDLY BAKING GUIDANCE

Simple ingredient substitutions and adjustments can help bakers with kidney disease meet their nutritional needs. For example, all-purpose flour can be substituted with lower-phosphorus and lower-potassium alternatives like almond or oat flour.

Egg whites can also be used in place of whole eggs to reduce phosphorus content while preserving texture and structure in baked goods. Finally, non-dairy milk like almond or coconut milk can also help lower the levels of phosphorus and potassium in recipes.

Kidney-friendly banana bread, for instance, can be made with almond flour, ripe bananas, and a small amount of honey or stevia for sweetness. This modification guarantees a tasty and moist dessert that complies with dietary restrictions.

In addition, baking fruits by grilling or poaching them instead of baking them at high heat retains their natural flavors and nutrients. These suggestions enable people to enjoy baked goods while putting their kidney health first.

TAKING CARE OF PHOSPHORUS IN SWEETS

Phosphorus control is important for people with kidney disease because high phosphorus can lead to heart and bone problems. Low-phosphorus ingredients such as unsweetened almond milk, oats, and fruits like apples or berries help keep the phosphorus balance in desserts. Baking powder also has less phosphorus than baking soda, so using it instead of baking soda lowers the amount of phosphorus consumed.

Here's a low-phosphorus chia seed pudding recipe that uses almond milk and fresh berries as the topping. Rich in fiber and omega-3 fatty acids, chia seeds provide extra health benefits while regulating phosphorus levels. Alternatively, a low-phosphorus dessert option is a sorbet made from blended frozen fruits and coconut water. By concentrating on phosphorus-conscious ingredients and preparation methods, people can enjoy desserts that support their kidney health goals without sacrificing taste.

DIALYSIS PATIENT RECIPES

Dialysis patients frequently need to make specific dietary adjustments to effectively manage their condition. It is important to select recipes that are high in essential nutrients and low in potassium, phosphorus, and sodium. For example, a kidney-friendly cheesecake made with tofu instead of cream cheese and a crust made with crushed almonds or oats offers a dessert option that is high in protein but low in phosphorus. Similarly, a salad of watermelon and cucumber dressed with lemon juice and fresh herbs offers a hydrating and refreshing dessert option.

Additionally, desserts such as baked pears stuffed with a cinnamon-ricotta cheese mixture provide a satisfying dessert without being overly high in potassium or phosphorus.

These recipes not only accommodate dietary restrictions but also encourage diversity and enjoyment in the diet of patients receiving dialysis. Through the exploration of inventive and nutrient-dense recipes, patients receiving dialysis can continue to enjoy delicious desserts without compromising their health.

TIPS FOR HYDRATION IN RENAL HEALTH

To maintain overall fluid balance and flush toxins from the body, proper hydration is essential. For renal patients, finding optimal hydration means balancing fluid intake with kidney function. First, follow your doctor's recommendations for fluid intake, which may differ based on your particular kidney health. Usually, this means limiting fluids if you have fluid retention or is on dialysis, but also making sure you drink enough to avoid dehydration.

It's equally important to choose the right fluids. Water is usually the best option because it has no calories, sugar, or additives. Herbal teas and infused water can add taste and variety without the added sugars that many other beverages contain. It's best to stay away from caffeinated and alcoholic drinks because they dehydrate the body. Instead, choose hydrating fruits and vegetables like watermelon, cucumber, and oranges to help meet your daily fluid needs.

For kidney health, it is imperative to maintain a low-potassium diet, particularly for patients with kidney disease who may have trouble eliminating potassium from their bodies.

When choosing drinks, go for low-potassium options to prevent your kidneys from being overworked. Some good options are apple juice, cranberry juice cocktail, and lemonade made with fresh lemon juice and sugar substitute.

Low-potassium drinks that can still be hydrating without compromising kidney function include coconut water and herbal teas like peppermint or chamomile. Be sure to always read labels to determine the potassium content of drinks, as some seemingly harmless beverages may have higher than normal levels. If your doctor hasn't specifically advised it, stay away from potassium-rich beverages like orange juice, tomato juice, and sports drinks.

Herbal teas and infusions provide a tasty substitute for regular beverages and are high in potassium and caffeine; for kidney patients, it's crucial to choose teas that are low in potassium.

Popular hot or cold herbal options include hibiscus tea, ginger tea, and rooibos tea; these teas not only hydrate but may also have health benefits like antioxidant and anti-inflammatory qualities.

Infusions, which involve soaking fruits or herbs in water to impart flavor, can also be a refreshing option. For example, a cucumber and mint infusion or a citrus peel and ginger infusion can provide a flavorful twist to your hydration routine without added sugars or artificial ingredients. To make herbal teas, steep the desired herbs in hot water for several minutes, then strain before drinking.

When made carefully with kidney-friendly ingredients, smoothies can be a nourishing and refreshing choice for patients on dialysis. Begin with a base of low-potassium fruits like berries, apples, or pears. Add a liquid base, such as almond milk or coconut water, which has a lower potassium content than dairy or regular fruit juices. Steer clear of using large amounts of potassium-rich fruits, like bananas or oranges.

Smoothies are a convenient way to hydrate and nourish your body while following kidney-friendly dietary guidelines. You can add nutritional value to your smoothie by blending in low-potassium protein powders or Greek yogurt (in moderation). You can also add a handful of spinach or kale for added vitamins and fiber, but be careful to keep potassium levels in check.

STEER CLEAR OF HIGH-SUGAR DRINKS

Avoiding high-sugar beverages is essential for kidney patients to maintain stable blood sugar levels and overall health. Sugary drinks, such as energy drinks, sodas, and sweetened teas, raise blood pressure, cause weight gain, and worsen the risk of diabetes, all of which can worsen the condition of their kidneys. Instead, choose sugar-free alternatives or drinks sweetened with artificial sweeteners, such as stevia or sucralose, but use them sparingly and consult your physician first.

You can effectively support your kidney health by reducing your sugar intake and making informed choices. Natural options, such as infused water with lemon or cucumber slices, can provide a refreshing alternative without added sugars. Diluted fruit juices and unsweetened herbal teas can also be enjoyed safely. When in doubt, carefully read nutrition labels to avoid hidden sugars and consult with a dietitian or healthcare provider for personalized recommendations.

CHAPTER FIVE

EATING OUT WHILE SUFFERING FROM KIDNEY DISEASE

When dining out, make sure to communicate your dietary restrictions to the server and ask about menu modifications. Choose grilled, baked, or steamed dishes instead of fried ones to reduce fat and sodium content. Request sauces and dressings on the side to control portions and avoid hidden sodium.

Planning is essential when dining out with kidney disease to maintain a balanced diet while managing sodium, potassium, and phosphorus intake.

Dining out with kidney disease can still be enjoyable and support your health goals if you plan and make informed choices. Take into consideration choosing meals with fresh vegetables and fruits that are lower in potassium and phosphorus. Steer clear of heavily processed, cured, or smoked dishes, as they often contain high levels of sodium and phosphorus.

Limit sugary drinks that can affect blood sugar levels and cause weight gain. Drink plenty of water or unsweetened beverages to stay hydrated.

TAKING CARE OF YOUR NUTRITION AND WEIGHT

Understanding your daily caloric needs based on your age, gender, activity level, and general health is the first step in managing your weight and nutrition. You should strive to incorporate nutrient-dense foods like fruits, vegetables, whole grains, and lean proteins into your diet while limiting processed foods, sugars, and saturated fats. Portion control is also crucial to prevent overeating and maintain a healthy weight.

A balanced diet, portion control, and regular physical activity are all important for managing weight, enhancing overall health, and supporting kidney function.

A registered dietitian can offer personalized guidance on developing a meal plan that satisfies your nutritional needs while taking into account the limitations imposed by kidney disease. Aim for at least 150 minutes of moderate-intensity exercise per week, such as brisk walking, swimming, or cycling.

Making educated decisions and adhering to a kidney-friendly diet requires that you effectively read food labels. To begin with, determine how much of the product you're eating by looking at the serving size. Next, consider the sodium content per serving, aiming for foods that have less than 140 milligrams per serving or selecting products labeled as "low sodium."

Finally, keep an eye on your potassium and phosphorus levels, preferring foods with lower amounts to preserve kidney function.

A dietitian can offer more advice on how to interpret food labels and choose products that support kidney health. By learning to read food labels, you can effectively manage your diet and support kidney health.

Look for labels that indicate "phosphorus additives" or "phosphate additives." Scan the ingredient list to identify additives and preservatives that may contribute to high sodium or phosphorus levels. Choose foods with natural ingredients and avoid those with added salts or phosphates.

SPEAKING WITH YOUR NUTRITIONIST

Your dietitian will evaluate your past eating habits, medical history, and kidney function to create a nutrition plan that supports optimal health. They will offer guidance on managing sodium, potassium, and phosphorus intake while ensuring adequate protein and nutrient levels. Regular consultations allow for adjustments based on changes in kidney function or health status. Speaking with a registered dietitian is essential to creating a personalized meal plan that is tailored to your needs if you have kidney disease.

By working with a dietitian, you can improve your dietary habits and overall well-being by learning about portion control, reading food labels, and making healthy choices both at home and when dining out. Dietitians can also address concerns about managing weight, controlling diabetes, and other health conditions that may affect kidney health. Regular follow-ups with dietitians ensure ongoing support and necessary meal plan adjustments, promoting long-term kidney health.

ADAPTING RECIPES TO DIALYSIS REQUIREMENTS

Modifying ingredients to meet dietary restrictions without sacrificing flavor and nutritional value is the first step in adapting recipes to dialysis needs. Herbs, spices, and citrus juices can be used as flavor enhancers instead of salt to lower sodium content. Tomatoes, bananas, and potatoes are examples of foods high in potassium; instead, choose lower-potassium options like apples, berries, and green beans. Lean protein sources like chicken, turkey, or fish and trim visible fat to lower phosphorus intake.

Whole grains like quinoa, brown rice, or whole wheat pasta can be added to meals to boost fiber intake and promote digestive health.

Portion control and weight management are important for dialysis patients, so try different cooking techniques like baking, grilling, or steaming to cut fat without compromising flavor. Speaking with a dietitian can offer more advice on how to adjust recipes and make meal plans that support the objectives of dialysis treatment.

CHAPTER SIX

PRACTICAL ADVICE AND LIFESTYLE TIPS

REMAINING ENGAGED DESPITE KIDNEY DISEASE

Maintaining a healthy weight, controlling blood pressure, and improving circulation are all critical for kidney function. However, it's important to choose activities that are easy on the body and steer clear of strenuous exercises that could strain the kidneys. Walking, swimming, and yoga are great examples of activities that provide cardiovascular benefits without unduly taxing the kidneys. As such, staying physically active is essential for managing kidney disease and promoting overall health.

It is crucial to speak with your healthcare provider before beginning any exercise program to make sure it is safe for your particular condition. They can provide customized exercise recommendations based on your overall health and kidney function. It is also important to stay hydrated while exercising because dehydration can exacerbate kidney function. You should also pay attention to your energy levels and listen to your body; if you feel tired or in pain, you should rest and modify your activity level accordingly.

Remember that maintaining an active lifestyle with kidney disease is not only good for your physical health but also for your mental health, making you feel more energized and optimistic about your overall health journey. Incorporating physical activity into your daily routine can be as easy as doing gentle stretches in the morning or taking short walks after meals. Setting realistic goals and gradually increasing your activity level can help you stay motivated and maintain consistency.

MANAGING NUTRITIONAL LIMITATIONS

The key to coping with dietary restrictions is knowing which foods are kidney-friendly and which ones to limit or avoid. A renal diet typically involves controlling protein, sodium, potassium, and phosphorus intake to support kidney function and prevent complications.

Living with kidney disease can make managing dietary restrictions difficult, but with careful planning and education, it is possible to enjoy a varied and nutritious diet.

Grocery shopping and meal preparation can be made easier by learning to read food labels and becoming familiar with substitute ingredients. For instance, selecting fresh produce with lower potassium levels, going for lean protein sources like fish or chicken, and substituting herbs and spices for salt can all help you make tasty, kidney-friendly meals. It's also critical to stay hydrated by drinking enough fluids throughout the day unless directed otherwise by your healthcare provider.

Finding new recipes and cooking techniques can make mealtimes more enjoyable and help you maintain a positive attitude toward your dietary restrictions. Speaking with family and friends about your dietary needs can help them understand and accommodate you when planning meals or dining out.

By being proactive and focusing on nutrient-dense, kidney-friendly foods, you can effectively manage your dietary restrictions and support your kidney health.

TIPS FOR DINING OUT AND SOCIALIZING

Socializing and going out to eat can both be enjoyable while following a renal diet if you plan. Before going out to eat, it's helpful to research which restaurants offer kidney-friendly options or can accommodate special dietary needs. Many restaurants will make dish adjustments upon request, such as lowering the salt content or switching to higher-potassium ingredients.

Focus on ordering simple preparations like baked or grilled dishes, and ask for sauces and dressings on the side to control portions. You can vary your meal without going overboard with a side salad dressed in vinaigrette or ordering steamed vegetables. It's also a good idea to let the restaurant staff knows exactly what you're eating so they can make sure your meal satisfies your nutritional needs.

When attending social gatherings that entail potlucks or meals at someone's house, think about bringing along a kidney-friendly dish to share. This way, you can be sure you have something to eat that is safe, and you can introduce others to tasty and nutritious options that complement your renal diet. Sharing your dietary restrictions with friends and family can help to build understanding and support, which will help to make socializing a positive experience that supports your health objectives.

ORGANIZING MEALS FOR EVENTS AND HOLIDAYS

It can be difficult to plan meals for holidays and special occasions, but with careful planning and inventiveness, you can enjoy celebratory times while adhering to your renal diet. To begin, make a meal plan that consists of kidney-friendly recipes and makes use of seasonal, lower-sodium, potassium, and phosphorus ingredients. This will keep you organized and prevent you from making impulsive decisions that might not be in line with your dietary requirements.

Offer to bring a dish that satisfies your dietary requirements when you attend events to make sure you have a healthy option that you can enjoy. Search for recipes that are flavorful and satisfying, like citrus-marinated grilled chicken skewers or roasted vegetables with herbs. Fresh fruits and salads can bring color and variety to the meal while providing essential nutrients.

To avoid misunderstandings and guarantee that the options available fit your renal diet, it's also helpful to let the host or hostess know in advance about your dietary requirements. You can also make sure that the options available fit your renal diet. Finally, remember to stay hydrated during the celebration by drinking water or other kidney-friendly beverages, and enjoy the celebration knowing that you've made choices that support your health goals.

MAINTAINING YOUR MOTIVATION DURING YOUR RENAL DIET

Long-term success and general well-being depend on your ability to stay motivated during your renal diet journey. Make realistic, attainable goals like cutting back on sodium gradually or experimenting with new kidney-friendly recipes every week. Acknowledge small victories along the way, like hitting milestones in your dietary goals or experiencing improvements in your general health and energy levels.

Seek out assistance from medical professionals, support groups, or online communities to connect with like-minded individuals managing kidney disease. Exchanging stories, advice, and encouragement can offer inspiration and a sense of community that you're not alone on this journey. Become knowledgeable about renal health and the advantages of a renal diet to strengthen your resolve and empower you to make wise decisions.

Try new flavors and cooking methods to make meals exciting and fun. Add diversity to your diet by trying foods from different cultures and seasonal produce that is naturally lower in potassium and phosphorus. Record your progress and changes in a journal or diary so you can look back on your accomplishments and overcome obstacles, which will inspire you to keep eating healthily.

You can stay motivated on your renal diet journey and make long-lasting adjustments that support your kidney health and general well-being by being proactive, finding help, and being informed.

CHAPTER SEVEN

MEETING YOUR NEEDS FOR PROTEIN

To provide essential amino acids without overtaxing the kidneys, it's important to meet your needs for protein, which requires careful balance. High-quality protein sources, like lean meats, eggs, and tofu, are recommended in moderate amounts; however, it's important to speak with a healthcare provider or dietitian to find out how much protein is appropriate for your particular condition, as protein needs can vary depending on the stage of kidney disease and whether you're on dialysis. Generally speaking, people with early-stage kidney disease may need to limit their protein intake, while those receiving dialysis may need to consume more because of the protein lost during treatments.

Aside from plant-based proteins like beans and lentils, which should be consumed in moderation due to their potassium and phosphorus content, protein can be incorporated into meals through creative cooking methods and portion control. For instance, you can add a small portion of grilled chicken or fish to a vegetable stir-fry to ensure that you're getting high-quality protein without excessive amounts. Recipes in the Kidney Disease Diet Cookbook frequently offer alternatives and modifications to balance protein intake effectively.

A food diary can help track protein consumption and ensure you're meeting but not exceeding your needs for protein. Regular check-ins with a dietitian can help adjust your diet as your condition changes, ensuring that your protein intake supports your overall health and kidney function. Monitoring protein intake involves not only choosing the right types of protein but also being mindful of portion sizes and meal frequency.

CONTROLLING FLUID CONSUMPTION

One of the most important parts of a kidney disease diet, particularly for dialysis patients, is controlling fluid intake.

Drinking too much fluid can lead to edema, hypertension, and dyspnea, while drinking too little can cause dehydration. The objective is to strike a balance between maintaining adequate fluid intake and preventing the kidneys from becoming overworked.

Effective strategies for managing fluid intake include measuring liquids and distributing fluid consumption throughout the day; sipping small amounts of water and using smaller cups can help with intake control; keeping an eye on the fluid content of foods is crucial; for example, selecting fruits with lower water content, like apples, over those with higher water content, like watermelon; ice chips can also be a useful way to quench thirst without consuming large amounts of liquid.

A journal or app can help you monitor your daily fluid intake and stay within your limits. Working with your healthcare team will ensure that your fluid management plan is customized to your unique needs and conditions, providing a safer and more comfortable approach to managing kidney disease. Flavor enhancers like lemon wedges or mint leaves can make limited fluid intake more satisfying and help reduce the temptation to drink more than the recommended amount.

ADVICE FOR PATIENTS RECEIVING DIALYSIS

Dialysis patients typically require higher protein intake, so including lean meats, fish, and egg whites in meals can help meet these needs. Keeping an adequate calorie intake is crucial to prevent weight loss and muscle wasting, and nutrient-dense foods like nuts, seeds, and healthy oils can help manage these unique dietary challenges. One important aspect is understanding the importance of a balanced diet that supports overall health and compensates for the nutrients lost during dialysis treatments.

Dialysis patients also need to control their potassium and phosphorus levels because high levels of these minerals can lead to major health problems. Low-potassium foods like cucumbers and green beans and high-potassium foods like bananas and oranges can help lower potassium intake, and low-phosphorus foods like almond milk can help lower phosphorus intake. It can be easier to do this by reading food labels and working with a dietitian to identify which foods to limit or avoid.

Hydration is another important area for dialysis patients because it's often necessary to restrict their fluid intake. Some practical strategies to help with this include measuring your intake, distributing fluids throughout the day, and using smaller cups to control consumption. You can also monitor your weight every day to help identify fluid retention early on and make necessary adjustments. Keeping a thorough food and fluid diary can help you keep track of your intake and maintain the delicate balance that proper dialysis management requires.

COMPREHENDING RENAL DRUGS

Renal medications are an essential part of managing kidney disease, and knowing their functions and interactions can improve their efficacy. These medications can include blood pressure control, diabetes management, cholesterol reduction, and anemia treatment. Since each medication has a unique mechanism of action, patients can better follow their treatment regimens if they understand it. For example, blood pressure medications such as ACE inhibitors not only lower blood pressure but also protect kidney function by lowering proteinuria.

Phosphate binders, for example, should be taken with meals to effectively reduce phosphate absorption from food. It is important to take medications exactly as prescribed and to be aware of potential side effects. Certain renal medications can cause side effects like dizziness, gastrointestinal problems, or electrolyte imbalances. Patients who are aware of these possibilities can recognize and report side effects promptly to their healthcare providers.

Keeping an updated list of all medications, including over-the-counter medications and supplements, can help prevent harmful interactions. Pharmacists can also provide valuable information on how to take medications correctly and what to do if a dose is missed. Effective management of renal medications requires regular communication with healthcare providers. Patients who understand the role and management of renal medications are empowered to take an active role in their treatment, which improves their overall health and quality of life.

HANDLING YOUR CRAVINGS FOR FOOD

Food cravings are a common challenge for people with kidney disease, but they can be managed with practical strategies. The first step is identifying the underlying cause of the cravings, which can be hunger, emotional triggers, or nutrient deficiencies. For example, cravings for high-potassium or high-phosphorus foods can often be mitigated by locating appropriate low-potassium or low-phosphorus alternatives. If you're craving salty foods like chips, try something small like air-popped popcorn or unsalted pretzels.

Eating a variety of flavors and textures in your diet can make meals more satisfying and reduce the desire for non-compliant foods. Fruits like berries or a small serving of applesauce can be a healthier choice that still satisfies the urge for something sweet. Planning meals and snacks ahead of time can also help manage cravings. Having kidney-friendly options readily available reduces the temptation to reach for foods that might be harmful.

An individual with kidney disease can better control their diet and maintain their health while still enjoying a variety of satisfying foods by practicing mindful eating, which involves eating slowly, savoring each bite, and paying attention to your body's hunger and fullness cues. It can also help identify true hunger versus emotional eating. Other strategies for managing cravings include staying hydrated, managing stress, and getting regular physical activity.